JUST PLAIN FAT

Just Plain Fat

Jeanne Cloutier-Fransway

To order additional copies of this book, contact:
Xlibris Corporation
1-888-795-4274
www.Xlibris.com
Orders@Xlibris.com
78110

To My Son, Tyler

The Joy and Love of My life

Well it has taken me 43 years and 10 months to realize that I needed to make a life change for my health. Some would say that is being lazy and others might say better now then never and I would like to choose the latter.

I have been heavy all my life and swore that I would never be that fat lady whose belly is to her knees and everyone looks and wonder how she got that fat. Well I became both of those things. We all know that it did not happen over night. So why would I let it happen? I use to cross country ski, dance, take 3-5 mile walks, and play some tennis here and there. In fact when I had to sell my ski's I cried. You would also think that being teased all the time and called names when you were younger would have left some impact to keep one's self from getting fatter. Being younger doesn't necessarily mean being a kid either. I was 21 when I was called Aunt Jemima. I still remember these as it were yesterday, so apparently the scars remain. Just because I am obese doesn't mean that I don't have feelings and for some odd reason some people just don't get that.

Basically it all comes down to years of excuses, mine being my health issues. My number one enemy is arthritis from an early age. And boy did I use that excuse to the hilt. I am not saying that there are not days that I could hardly move nor did I not want to move, which is most of them. I had a very bad knee that did not allow me to do much but to work. But I was old enough and smart enough to know better. No body knows better than a fellow suffer of arthritis how easy it is to chose not to move because you can move so little most of the time.

So now the saga begins of the journey of weight gain. You start feeling that you are dammed if you do and dammed if you don't. By that I mean you are too sore and stiff to exercise and if you got on the floor you would never get up again or need a crane to get you standing up. So now you have acquired the attitude that it doesn't matter you can't move to exercise so you are stuck at where you are at. So the whole concept of exercising is now something that is not even a thought process any more, it doesn't exist to you any more. Then comes the issue of eating. Did I watch what I ate since I didn't exercise? You bet I did, I watched everything that went into my mouth, every bite at a time, pound after pound, year after year, and chocolate bar after chocolate bar.

I can tell you that being fat, obese, over weight or what ever nice word you want to name it is no picnic. Fat is fat. To the world that is not over weight I often wonder does that sector of society ever wonder what our world is like. Do they even know of all the problems that fat causes besides the obvious health issues. Do we as fat people even realize these issues are self or do we just accept them and try to do the best that one can? I am not writing these issues to be gross or funny, it is a fact in the fat world. I want people to know the real truth about being fat and not just hear what they want to hear or think about fat people.

You go to a restaurant and you hope and pray that they have chairs without arms or that you don't have to squeeze yourself into a booth and hope that you can get back out without taking the booth table out with you at the same time. If that does happen you are hoping that the restaurant isn't very busy and no one noticed. When eating out, you see people looking at you and then talking so now you don't even enjoy your meal any more because of all the things that are going through your head about what they are saying about you. Or if you are at an office some where and you have to sit side ways on your hip to sit in the little chair with arms and hope that the chair doesn't sick to your ass when you get up or even break. Or to even avoid some of this I would find myself calling ahead some where to request that there be a chair available with no arms to even avoid the embarrassing issue. Or when the little boy in the grocery store says, "hey why are you so fat?" A good question I would say. This is just the tip of the iceberg so to speak of things that happen in public not to mention the things that go on in the home.

This one was never an issue for me, not being able to wipe your butt, because your arms and hips are too fat to reach back there. But believe me I had other issues. My legs are beet colored with blue spider veins for decorations. Then on the days with water pooling at my ankles it looked like I was walking on poorly decorated stumps. With the weight and being stiff and one artificial knee I could hardly get socks on and could hardly get a shoe on. On those days that I needed to wears these I thank God for my son to help me get dressed.

Then there is the issue of cloths. Lucky for me I can sew and could make myself some very nice dresses. But in reality they were still all one size bag fits all, just some nice material that could hang over the fat. Under garments are a whole another issue in them selves. There are none that fit with any dignity.

Bathing was never an issue for me either, but I have heard that some people have to have help with that also. But there definitely is the issue of skin sores and break down from any little moisture being trapped in some dark hidden skin folds. Sometimes when a sore would appear under some fold or the other, I would think that I had more folds than a Sharpie dog. So haul out every kind of powder, deodorant, and cream that would help keep those areas dry, sore free and God for bid odor free.

I am not sure what it is like for other heavy people, but for me I think that I was like an anorexic on the opposite side of the mirror. I never saw myself as that fat. I knew that I was fat but never felt like I was as fat as I was. My brain wasn't fat just me. The whole time of being fat I never once have seen myself as being ugly either. I think that I am not bad looking other wise. It has never been an issue of low self esteem either for me. But there are other issues that one can use their fat to hide behind. Any expert can give you pages of them. For me I think, no not think, I know it is that I always wanted the marriage that my husband would love me forever and grow old with me for better or worse or fat. That dream ended in divorce. So for me if I stayed fat no one would want me so then I would not have to feel that kind of loneliness, no one to share things with and yes sex. Because I resolved myself to the fact that I am alone and single. So with that thought of thinking I can't feel alone.

So where or what in one's life makes the difference to take the first steps to change? It has been something that has been in the back of my mind for a long time that I needed to do something about it, but just didn't act upon it. My son's godmother asked me to be in her wedding and that even really wasn't the motivator because in my head I knew that I would have to opt out because I won't be able to find a dress to fit. So for me it was a TV show called Nip and Tuck. This is quite funny since I don't really watch that much TV in the first place. They aired a show about a very obese woman who spent three years on her couch who literally did not move from that couch. I swore that night that I would not be that fat lady on the couch hauled away on a fire truck flat bed to the hospital.

The next day I ordered a tread mill and started thinking about how I was going to change my life forever. It wasn't going to be just a diet. Dieting is to lose a few pounds so that you can fit into your Christmas dress. I had even entertained the idea of a stomach by pass.

I needed to be exercising and eating right for the rest of my life. So now once again the hard journey begins to lose all that fat. My life now consists of diet scales, measuring cups, reading labels, and planning meals. Drinking lots of water or tea because one doesn't want to waste their calorie intake on juices. Here is where I wish that I was wealthy and could hire a chef to deal with the meals, and calorie counting. The grocery bill has gone up since it is more expensive to eat healthy. It really is a shame that a head of cauliflower cost about the same amount as three boxes of macaroni and cheese. No wonder the nation as a whole is getting fatter.

My new best friend is a black tread mill which is set up in the living room so there are no excuses not to use it. We have a date five days a week for a half hour getting in a little over a mile. But getting to that half hour is very difficult at best and very hard work for me. My feet and hips like to cramp up on me and I have to stop, rest, and work the cramps off just to get back on to get that half mile in. Some days it takes an hour to get that half hour in. It was no easy feat to get up to a half hour. Talk about baby steps. The first time was two and half minutes and I thought for sure I was going to die. I was huffing and puffing and hurt like hell. Then it was three minutes three times a day. Then I made it to five minutes three times a day and so on. It took me two and half weeks to get up to that half hour. There are days when I am walking that track watching animal planet (I decided to get educated while walking) that I keep thinking God I wish I didn't have to do this. So as I am sweating now with a raised heart rate, sore feet, and hips, I pray real hard for God to give me strength to continue and thank him when I reach that last minute to go. I also thank him every week when I step on that scale and see that my life changes are paying off. I also thank my family and friends for their continued support on this new journey.

12/24/2005

Well it is now two months into my new journey and I have to come to three definite conclusions; one I envy people who are skinny with no effort. Secondly it is easier just being fat. There is no effort or discipline being fat, it just happens. Thirdly sugar is the root of all evil. I had decided that on New Year's Eve that it would be my cheat day and I would see the year 2005 out with a bang. I sure did. I over ate on New Year's Eve with Christmas goodies like fudge, cookies, etc. By doing that I brought the New Year in with an extreme headache, sick to my stomach and feeling just plain yucky. Another lesson learnt; eat in moderation!

There is no other goal in life that has more discipline and dedication then a fat person wanting to become a thin person. Now I have to get up and exercise whether I want to or not because the fat isn't going to fall off by it's self. Yet I think it should be by now by how hard I am working. Some days looking at the tread mill it would be so easy to say that I did it, but didn't. Eating healthier really is the easy part in all this. Once you get use to eating the right way and you eat crap for a day for what ever reason you pay for it by feeling like crap. My body really feels good and likes the healthier eating. I have found that it doesn't matter when you eat or why you eat something, it is what you eats that matters.

I was hoping by now that my flat feet would be a little forgiving, but no go. Not sure what I was expecting with cocked and twisted toes with the cartilage pulled off a couple of them. But one can hope.

I did gain three pounds over the Holidays which isn't too bad. Which makes me wonder how many pounds will I lose and lose again because I decide to eat unhealthy. I did lose them again with another pound, so I have lost 33 pounds and 15 inches which has put me into one size smaller dress. Not only am I using the tread mill now I have also joined Curves. At this point I am still not sure how working on a machine for 30 seconds, jumping on a board and moving on to the next machine is really going to help, but only time will tell. I am stiffer at night and in the morning since starting this new activity.

A big mile stone in my new journey, I am wearing a pair of jeans and a T-shirt, something I haven't been able to do for many years. The T-shirt is actually loose. The other day I spent a few hours reacquainting myself with some clothes in my closet.

Well it has turned out that Curves was not the thing for me right now, but maybe later. It really threw my arthritic joints for a curve no pun intended. I could hardly move my shoulders, and my low back was the worse.

Today is January 13, 2006 and is my 44th birthday and my goal was to have off 40 pounds by today. I fell two pounds short. When I stepped on the scale this AM it was the first time that I was very emotional and started crying. I am not really sure what the tears were for or why. I do know that for the first time on this new journey I felt an accomplishment. My friends and family are so supportive. They tell me all the time how proud of me they are. My mom and Aunt Dee tell everyone about me and how I am changing my life.

There has been a little set back on the tread mill. I was up to 2.4 miles per hour walking and due to my poor flat arthritic feet I started getting shine splits and had to drop down to 2.2 miles per hour. But it took care of the problem with the shins. I sure was hoping that with time the exercising would get easier. But my feet and hips still like to cramp up and it still takes me an hour some times to get my half hour in on the tread mill.

As we all know in life there a set backs here and there for what ever the reasons. This time it is surgery on my right elbow. This surgery took a lot more out of me than I had planned and hoped for. The pain control was the biggest issue. It has taken a lot of pain meds to keep me comfortable, so I slept and rested a lot. It has been three days since I have done the tread mill and I do not like how I am feeling. It is almost like I can feel the weight slowly ounce by ounce to start to creep up on me even though I am still eating right. It really is funny if you think about how when starting out one doesn't really like the idea of exercising let alone doing it and jokes about how the tread mill is now their new best friend. When in reality it has become your true new best friend. It never let's you down and it always there for you and makes you feel good about yourself. So I hit the tread mill and was only able to do eleven and a half minutes. I was happy with that because it was better than nothing and I know with a little patience and time I will be right back where I was. Well the next day I got twenty three minutes in through out the day. The next day I was right back on track with thirty minutes.

Earlier in my journey of being fat I talked about how we as fat people just accept the things that we can or can not do because of our weight or do not realize that what ever it is we are doing is difficult. For example the other day my son made a comment that I sure can get into his truck easier now that I have lost some weight. It was only at that moment I realized that he was right and had never paid attention to it. So it made me to start to think about other things that have become easier, not even counting the increase energy level. Simple things like bending over, putting shoes on, being able to scratch somewhere you haven't been able to reach before. All the little things that we as humans just accept and take for grant it, fat or not.

On this journey I have read and researched so many of the diet plans out there from Jenny Craig, Weight Watchers, Atkins, Denise Austin,

The Zone, and I could go on and on there is so many. I have also bought some of the so called "Magic Pills", Green tea, Insta Ultra Trim, Miracle Burn, Carbs by Jake just to name a few to see what was in these items to make people think that these would help them burn fat. The most common element in most of these items is Chromium. There are also items like the Patch, Electrical Muscle Stimulators, and the Miracle Juice. There was also some item that my sister was telling me about that she put in her ear and was suppose to rub when she got hungry. She said that all she got was a sore ear. I am not able to say that these items do not work for people to help them on their way to weight loss. These items do mention in fine print that one needs to exercise and eat better. But they also make it sound like that by just taking this product you will lose weight with out any effort. A fat's person dream! One cannot truly believe that sitting in front of the TV, eating chips and taking a "magic pill" is going to help them burn off the fat. Because if there really was that "Magic Pill" that melted your fat away while you slept the whole world would be thin. There would be no such thing as obesity, diet programs, diet aids, dieticians, and gyms. The diet industry has become a master in creating fantasy fixes with false hopes. Not one of these products has been effective in healthily long term permanent weight loss. So despite all the claims made by these companies there is no easy fix. It all comes down to the true basic facts of eating right, exercising, and taking control of our lives.

My little sister has joined me on my journey and it was very exciting for me when she called and told me that she lost six pounds her first week and one size in clothes. To hear that excitement in her voice was so great. Now I know how proud she felt when I would call her with a fat loss up date. We talk just about every day, but now our talks also include sharing new recipes, what foods make a balanced block, how good we feel and the support that we give each other to continue with our new life styles. It is also so fun sharing the excitement together.

Well the first plateau has arrived! I am stuck at 36-38 pounds. Of course there are a couple factors here that may come into play thou. First off this last week and a half I have had to eat small healthily snacks when taking my pain pills so that I would not get stomach upset. Secondly I haven't been drinking water like I should either. Then God bless my son because he says "hey Mom it just might be water gain and not fat." Even so I have had to change some things like increasing my activity. It is hard doing that right now because my elbow really hurts and the walking does bother it believe it or not. So I have managed five more minutes in the morning and any where from five to fifteen minutes in the evening depending on the pain level. I have to be honest here and say that I am feeling a little depressed with this. I started losing weight like gang busters and then a dead stop. I have read so many articles about other people losing large amounts of weight in a short time and do not see that happening here with me. So I keep telling myself that I deserve to be thinner and just be patient it will start again.

Today January 30th, now 12 weeks later onto my journey I weighed in at 40 pounds lighter. I am so excited. I was saying yes, yes, at the scale when one of the nurses said, "it must be good news" and I said, that I hit the 40 pound mark and all three nurses said, "great job." It made me feel like I should run home and hop on the tread mill. I feel so good about myself that I can't wait to keep losing more.

I also need to mention here that The Zone way of eating is how I am accomplishing this weight loss with exercise. I decided on the Zone because so many of the other diets out there I have failed at. With the Zone you can eat what ever you want as long as the blocks are balanced. You can have your cheat day or meal and when you eat the next Zone meal you are right back on track. When eating balanced blocks you are not hungry or feel the need to have to eat. The Zone also has great bars and they fill that need to have something sweet once in a while.

January 31st and I went nineteen minutes at one time on the tread mill before my feet and hips started to cramp. This is the longest time at one stretch that I have been able to go. Another small feat for some people, but a big one for me.

I need to talk about some things that may be gross to talk about or some may even find it funny. But it is a fact that fat people can have a hard time wiping their butt. I was so ecstatic that I was now able to wipe my behind sitting on the toilet and did not have to stand up to do it. I found myself laughing and thinking how excited I was to be able to do a "normal" body function that I am sure for the most part society takes for grant it and never thinks about it for one minute. I was thinking of the automatic toilets that flush when you stand up. As a heavy person you stand up to wipe and then the toilet flushes so when you are done wiping you stand there like a flagman waving your arms around trying to get the toilet to flush again. Another accomplishment that may seem trivial to the average person, but the other day when I was at the doctor's office I sat with my butt flat in the chair and not on my hip to fit in the chair. Also when I stood up my butt didn't stick to the chair either. I found it quite interesting that this particular doctor who had read my journal so far made the comment that heavy people aren't really that happy and that they just want to fit in the "norm" of things. How true because just the fact that I could sit in an office waiting room chair like a "normal" person made me happy. Also when talking with this doctor I made the comment that fat people are stereo typed. He asked why? This particular doctor is very handsome and fit looking and I got the feeling that he really couldn't grasp what it would be like being fat. For the most part people think that just because we are fat that we are lazy and sit around all day doing nothing. I know this first hand because of a job that I once held.

One of the managers did not like hiring heavy women because of this way of thinking. Here I need to mention that I feel that obese women are more discriminated against then obese men.

There are so many incorrect assumptions about fat people and their life styles. Not all heavy people sit around eating Bon Bons and watching TV. Not all heavy people have large appetites as some may think. In fact when I was younger my mom would get so mad because she would watch me talk myself out of eating, when I should have been eating. In high school I ate a salad everyday for lunch just so the fat cells weren't chasing me down the hall to class. I would have much preferred to have been eating other things, but was too afraid of being teased about what I was eating.

Heavy people are not all sedentary as some may think.

In fact people who know me, know that I am a very busy person and is always doing something. I have never been a person who could just sit. It is very difficult for me to even just sit through a movie. It drives my son nuts because I am up and down all the time. He'll say, "Can't you just sit still relax and enjoy the movie?"

Yesterday the Zone emailed me and stated that they might have my success story featured on their website. I sent them my journals of becoming fat to try and win some cook books. Just being considered is an honor and a great motivator. At this point it is so hard not to keep talking about how great I feel about myself and how great my body is starting to feel. I no longer have that fat bloated feeling, or that mental feeling of fat. Which is a hard one to explain, but fellow obese people know what I am talking about. I really don't believe it is a depressed feeling at all, but I think the easiest way to explain it is that you have gotten to the point that you can't kid yourself anymore when you say that I am happy it doesn't matter that I am fat. With me I also kept telling myself that I have really bad arthritis so I won't be able to do things any way even if I was thinner. Now I keep thinking of all the things that will be easier and all of the things that I can try to do. I know that with the arthritis I will still have to be careful and do things in moderation, but I feel like I have a new chance at things that I deserve. Sitting here writing this I am crying. These tears are for all the things that I cheated my self out of because of not taking control of my life sooner. I know that with my arthritis that there are things that I won't have been able to do any way. But I do know with the weight there could have been things that maybe I would have been able to do in moderation with out difficulty. One of the greatest things I really regret is that I wasn't able to be the mom I wanted to be when my son was little. In my mind I wanted to be the mom that played ball, wrestled on the floor and played tag in the back yard. Things that I will have never done. I have been so blessed that I have a son that had never once growing up said things about my weight. He has truly loved me unconditionally for who I am and not what I could have been. Maybe if he had said something I might have taken control sooner. I hope that with my life changes that he will see that he also needs to take control of his weight. But as we all know that young teenagers think that they have time for everything and that they are invincible.

I am now down 45 pounds and 20 inches in thirteen weeks! I know this is a lot of weight, yet some times I feel like Dr Jekyll and Mr. Hyde. Some days I see myself as that thin person not as fat as I really am and other days all I see is the fat. I have noticed now at 45 pounds that I am starting to get some wrinkles on my face around my mouth and eyes. I have been doing the facial exercises where you form the vowels. Sure hope that these work. I don't want to look like I have aged. I would hate to have this new image and then look like a droopy old basset hound. I am sure this is one of many issues of skin that I will have to deal with. I can't expect my skin to be nice and firm when I have stretched it so badly over the years. I have also started to get some bags of skin hanging on my thighs, but at least that is in an area that I don't have to worry about people seeing. My neck and arms are also getting fine wrinkles now too. This is an issue that I am really concerned about. I know that when I reach my goal that my doctor and I have already discussed surgery. So I just have to keep telling myself that it will be okay and it will look better in the end, once again just be patient.

A couple weeks back I was able to wear one of my son's fleece pull overs. The look on his face was priceless. He just stood there and went ah, ah and I said "what?" He said nothing and just continued to stare at me. I asked him what was wrong and he said, "It is just funny seeing you in my clothes, the next thing I'll know you'll be wearing my jeans." "Good idea." I said. So then a couple days later there was a new fleece that I had purchased for him sitting on the table when he came home from school. As always he said "thanks Mom" and then he turns to me and says "or is this for you now?" I started laughing and said, "You know that I don't wear those colors of green." "Well I thought I should ask now that you are wearing my size." He says. It made me smile. He still is not too keen on the idea of me wearing his jeans thou. He keeps telling me that they won't fit me right and that I will most definitely have to get women's jeans. I think that is his way of drawing the line of what he will let me get away of wearing what is his.

As I sit here writing this I can't even begin to describe how bad I want the weight off. I am not a very patient person, I always want things done right now, if not yesterday. So it is going to be very hard, no difficult for me to be patient with this weight loss. For me it won't come off fast enough. I will have to keep telling myself that good things come to those who wait and that the hard work will pay off. God has tried teaching me patience, but this will be the ultimate lesson of learning those patience's. It really doesn't seem fair that the weight goes on so easy and them comes off so hard.

When reading articles in the past about women who have lost weight I always thought it was funny that in the after pictures they had changed their hair color and style. I would always think why do they do that? Now I know why. I am also in the process of changing my hair color. One it has to do with the new image and secondly for me to help hide the grey. It is all about the CHANGE. I keep thinking of all the things that I want to change with this new life style. My hair, my glasses to a new hip style or maybe even contacts again, my clothes, and wearing make up. Starting to use a good cleaning system for my face, all things that I want to do for me because I deserve it and it feels so good.

Went shopping for the first time for some new clothes since the weight loss and wasn't really sure what size I was going to be into. It ended up that I bought a pair of jeans that was a size 30, which were three sizes smaller. My bra size has gone from a 56 to a 48. I was also looking for some new causal dresses, and this particular store that I buy my clothes at has decided that they were no longer going to carry this item. I got very upset about that and then one of my friends reminded me that if would not matter because I will be able to buy my clothes at other stores now. It hadn't even crossed mind that I have now opened up another new world for myself by being able to buy clothes else where. It was a very exciting concept for me. I was ecstatic just thinking about it, let alone going out and doing it. It will be fun to shop and try on new clothes and not have it be the painful nightmare it use to be for me. Not to come home crying inside and depressed because I couldn't find anything. Then it also got me started thinking about all the clothes that I will be able to make and not have to enlarge the pattern any more. I literally have 100's of patterns and my mind was racing just thinking of all the cool dresses that I could start making myself because I really enjoy wearing dresses. It is also a good thing that I can sew because than I won't have to spend a lot of money during all the different size changes. I also took one of my dresses and packed it away last night. As I was folding it up and placing it in the drawer I was crying and saying this is my fat dress and you will always be here as a gentle reminder that I can always pull out to see my accomplishments.

Well this journey has opened so many different doors already that I get quite excited wondering what other new and different things will happen for me. One new and different thing is opening my self up to try different foods that I would have never considered before like spinach. I made it with broccoli and carrots in a garlic sauce and was very surprised that it was something that I would eat again.

Another thing that I have noticed on the health issue of this journey is that my legs no longer look that beet red color from poor circulation. My right leg that had a blood clot at one time is till darker in color and may always be that way. But they don't look like fat lady legs any more and plus the added bonus is that they now have shape to them from walking.

It is Monday and WOW what a horrible, horrible weekend! I am not sure why but all I wanted to do is eat. It was like a munchies attack. I ate good things like I am suppose to, but it was all weekend long. So now I feel awful physically and mentally. I feel bloated and icky.

But I think the mental part is really making me feel the worse. Because even thou we are educated human beings our minds are a double edge sword that keeps cutting out the logic and letting the negative in with the quilt. At least I know that I can get right back on track and haven't completely fallen off the wagon here. I want to go weigh myself to see what the damage is, but yet do I really want to know and then give myself more guilt over it. Or just wait, work out real hard this week and weigh myself on Friday. I think that I will opt for the latter.

I went to the beauty shop today to get my hair done. Which by the way I really like being a frosted blonde again. When I went to the beauty shop before my beautician always got out the folding chair for me because I did not fit in the regular salon chairs. Well guess what, I fit in the salon chairs now. There was no squishing into it; I just sat in it like everyone else does. Also why I was there I over heard another client talking about her diet. Then I heard her say that the weight just doesn't want to come off, but at least I am healthy. I had to chuckle, because we really are not healthy. Are poor bones and joints are stressed to the max. Our hearts and arteries are working over time, which usually causes us to have high blood pressure, our labs such as cholesterol, blood sugars, and so much more are often very high. Thus all these things predispose us to things such as stroke, heart attacks, and diabetes more than the average weight person.

I am happy to announce that my son has began asking me questions how he can reduce calories. Now I hope that he acts on it.

Well I ended up weighing in on Tuesday instead of Friday and I was shocked that after my munchies weekend binge that I had lost a pound, now making it 48 pounds total.

It is the weekend again and today is going to be a test for me. My friends are having pot luck for supper. I plan on eating what ever I want for my cheat meal of the week. But I just have to remember to eat in moderation and hope that the cheesy hash browns and the bacon broccoli salad don't call my name out to loudly. Well the cheesy hash browns and bacon broccoli salad did call my name for a second round, but both servings were small. I ate all good things and did not end up feeling like crap. So I feel that I mastered this pot luck quite nicely and have made another hurdle knowing that I have learned to eat in moderation. To other people this means nothing, but to me it is so funny that I actually want the good food over the junk food considering that I was a junk food junkie when it came to chips and dip. The other day I found myself looking for fruit over the bread. Also yesterday at the pot luck I was looking for the salad, where before I would have never given it a thought. Also since being on the Zone I no longer crave sweets or chocolate. Before the Zone it was like sweets and chocolates ruled me. There wasn't a day that didn't go by where I had some form of chocolate and had to have something sweet after a meal. I even had some form of chocolate stashed in the cupboard and believe me it yelled out my name so loud at times that I could hear it calling my name all the way down the hall into my bedroom at night.

I am also happy to announce that since eating right and exercising I do not hurt as much any more. In fact some days now I hardly notice the pain, which is something that hasn't happened in years.

I have gained three pounds in three days and I am panicking. I am still eating right and I have increased my walking to 35 minutes in the morning and ten minutes at night when tolerated. My clothes still continue to get looser thou. I am just hoping for some reason that it is water or muscle gain.

Well it has been water gain THANK GOD. Not sure why there is a problem with that thou. I don't use salt and I eat fresh fruit and vegetables. So I am still hanging on to those 49 pounds. Since there has been no scale movement I measure myself and I have lost another four inches, making it a total of twenty four inches now.

Tried a new recipe from the Zone cook book and was very impressed how good it tasted. Bought some tofu that I will have to get brave here in a couple days and try it.

My left knee which I call my good knee has started to catch, snap, and hurt. That really has me worried because I need to be able to use the tread mill; it has become my life line for me. So I have had to back down the speed once again and go a little slower. My arthritis is sure making this new journey more difficult. If I couldn't use the tread mill on account of my knee I don't know what I would do. I know in my heart that it is the exercise that is keeping the weight off. So I pray to God that it is his will not to have my knee go out on me, but that this is just his way of letting me know that I need to back off a little.

This last week I am happy to announce that I have noticed that my son has cut back on his eating.

Went to the doctor for my knee and got a cortisone injection which has helped with the pain, but no go with the snapping and cracking. Took x-rays and the doctor was really happy with them stating that there is a few more years of wear yet. I am looking at them and thinking Oh Shit. They are awful looking; bone space is very limited with bone on bone. Bone spurs on both sides of the knee and of course arthritis every where. It is my new life style that has set this bout off. But as we all know that I can't use it as an excuse not to exercise. So as long as I can walk, the tread mill it is. I will have to keep modifying as I go along. So I know I will probably have to decrease the speed and shorter periods at one time through out the day to get my half hour in. My doctor also said just keep on what your doing and don't stop because of it. Then to top it off I seen my mother's knee x-rays a few days later and I was jealous. Our x-rays should be turned around for our ages.

Been on a plateau now for over three weeks and I can see why people give up and say, "what is the use?" It is very disappointing and a little depressing, because you are still doing everything right. When one is at this point it is funny how the scale becomes your focal point. Being the humans that we are we focus on the negative and forget the positive things. We need to focus on the whole picture such as losing inches, feeling good and having more energy.

The good thing is that I have only fluctuated between two and three pound which tells me I am still on track, because of water weight changes going on. I know that it is just my body adjusting to all the changes and things will move again evidently. Once again I need to remind myself, patience my girl.

Just an added note here that from all the negative comments about tofu I haven't gotten the nerve up yet to try it. It has become the bottom of the food chain for me now. But I am going to start making soy protein smoothies for breakfast.

Well today I weighed in and the plateau is over at 51 pounds. I was so happy that I cried and was hugging my mom. The dietician and the nurse that was there were very impressed and started asking how I did it. When talking with them and telling them how it is a life style change, but it is also a mental change as well. Your heart and soul with your attitude have to be in this change together or it won't make any difference. Because if you don't have one with out the other you won't be able to deal with the obstacles that come with the life style change and weight loss. You would be only setting your self up for failure.

They were both very impressed and congratulated me. After talking with the dietician she told me that I would be perfect for a job in teaching weight management. I was impressed with that. This was such a joyous day for me, a fourth of the way to my goal in four months. I was so happy that once we got into the elevator I could not contain myself any more and did the happy dance.

Since being on this plateau I have noticed that I am more in tuned to my body. Without even looking at the scale I could feel that I wasn't losing weight. I can now feel again that I am losing. My body feels different in each one of these phases. I can actually feel when my body is in and out of the Zone. This is great for me because it really helps keep me on track. I like how my body feels when it is in the Zone.

Not sure how often this will happen but for the first time I went the full thirty minutes on the tread mill without stopping. The last eight minutes was done with a lot of praying and had to slow the speed down some, but I did it. Another feat for me, the other day I went 53 minutes total for the day on the tread mill. It feels good to be able to get more time in, but I also have to be careful because I feel okay when I am doing it, but then at night or the next day my knee is cracking and popping more and I will feel stiffer as a whole.

This is where and why it is so important that your mind and soul are together in this journey. So that when these obstacles come up, your mind will keep telling you that you are doing okay while your heart is saddened. I am having problems with water weight issues which keep showing up on the scale as gains. I know that when I gain two pounds in two or three days that it is water, but it is still disheartening, when you are looking forward to the scale going down. The weight coming off now is at a snail's pace and a geriatric snail with a cane at that. Patience, patience it will come off I keep telling myself.

The tread mill had been a lot easier this last week. I have been able to go longer at one time and do about 53 minutes a day now. I am really happy how much easier the tread mill had become this last two weeks. I am able to do about 40-45 minutes in less than an hour now most days. Depending on how I feel really regulates how much time I do each day. So some days it is more but never less than a half hour. My feet and hips are cramping a lot less and not so intense. What it really comes down to is the arthritis is the one in control of how long I walk and at what intensity. But it will never take total control again. I will do what ever modifying it takes to continue exercising.

I find it really funny how food centered our culture is and how everything seems to be associated with food. We eat when we are sad, when we are happy, bored, and some eat just to eat. We bribe our children with food to behave. My family and friends are comparing my weight loss to food items, for example someone had said just think you have loss 53 pounds and all I see is 53 pounds of hamburger, or two twenty five bags of potatoes, flour just to name a few.

YEAH, March 30, 2006 and I weighed in today at 55 pounds. Thank you God for your help in teaching me on this journey that patience, self control, and discipline are the keys to my success. With these three keys, God, my family and friends I can do anything that I put my mind too and get what I want.

Yesterday I announced to my family and friends that I hit the 55 pound mark and the next day my mom, friends Bernie, Shelby and Wendy came over to my house and brought me a beautiful humming bird sun catcher with a nice card to show there support, congratulations, and happiness for me. They will never know what their continued support and love means to me. I know that I am not on this journey by myself and that a lone makes it so much easier. I tried my fat dress on for them and they could not believe it when they actually saw it for themselves. Actually for me it is quite amazing also when I put it on and to realize that I filled that dress to where the buttons were pulling apart. Also showed them the new black dress that I bought that is smaller and will fit into soon. It was the first time today that I admitted out loud to anyone that even thou I like wearing dresses the fact was it was the only thing that fit over the fat. The only piece of clothing that didn't cut into me somewhere. Before when doing laundry all I had to do was pull out my dresses and the rest was my son's clothes. Now I have to sort through it because I now have jeans and shirts in there too. This makes me smile.

On this journey I find myself smiling a lot over the little things. Just everyday things that are considered "normal" or things that we take for grant it. The gift of life and the ability to live it is such a blessing. We need to embrace it, make every day count and run with it. Take what ever obstacles get in the way and learn from them. To know that you can be in control of your life and make the decisions that you need to be healthy and happy physically, mentally, emotionally and spiritually.

I am finding with this new life style that the biggest obstacle besides the arthritis is this dam up and down of water weight gain. It is very depressing to know that you are doing everything right and yet there is a three to four pound weight gain. It is so frustrating that it leaves this sense of doubt in what you are doing. May be the doctor will have some suggestions when I go and have my labs done this week. I can't wait to see if the numbers have changed at all. In the past I would dread my lab checks.

All my life when I was dieting and would eat something like cookies, candy etc, I would think well I might as well eat them all so they won't be there to tempt me the next day. Well lo and behold this way of thinking has a name for it. It is called "what the hell effect." You have your binge of three or four cookies and then you think, what the hell I have already blown it, so I might as well eat the whole dam box now. This way of thinking has gotten better for me with learning self control and portion control. Also learning not to over react and thinking that I have failed but have had just a momentary lapse of self control. Just get back on tract with the right foods and I will be just fine.

I find myself watching people eat now when I am out. This is something that I have never done before. I am now curious what people are eating. I could cringe at what I am seeing and I can hear their arteries screaming at them. Now I know what my sister means when she said that she would be so sad when she would watch me pack in the food. Our society is out of control with portions. Everywhere you go it is bigger size this bigger size that. Restaurants serve steaks that are half of the cow; bakeries make muffins the size of Frisbees. Society as a whole we are not satisfied unless our plates are over flowing and we get our monies worth. So that is where the doggie bag comes into play. Society could lose weight on average just by cutting their portions. This is something I have finally mastered on this journey and feel quite comfortable with. I now have an excellent eye and can tell just by looking at a piece of meat how many ounces it is.

Weighed in this morning and I tried so hard not to cry. I am up six pounds! I have to keep telling myself that the scale is not the true indicator of my success. The best measurements are; how do I feel and look? How are my clothes fitting? Just by exercising and eating right is success in it's self. Yet the scale still holds the most weight (no pun intended) when measuring our loss and giving us the feed back to measure that success with. A piece of metal with numbers now has the control to play havoc with our (my) emotions. My entire mood can be changed from this beastly piece of equipment which can make or break my day. I can be feeling so great and then when I see the numbers I can be totally devastated and made to cry. It can build us up or tear us down. So here is where my intelligence takes over and tells me that a scale should only be used as a guiding tool. The scale doesn't tell the whole story. It doesn't tell the life style changes you have made. There is no way that it can show that your body is becoming healthier and under going changes. It can not show the changes in your labs. Which by the way I need to add here that mine have gone down again in three months and are now normal for the first time in many years. So I need to just remember that the scale is only there to show a number and that the scale is not my best friend in the whole picture of things. Fluctuations are normal for what ever reasons and I need to take them in stride. I need to continue measuring my success with my attitude, how my clothes feel on me, feeling smaller, and the most rewarding is the comments made by friends and family on how good I am looking. Being told I look great is the reminder that my efforts of changing my life style are worth it and working.

The doctor is changing my medication to see if it will help with the water issues. Took a diuretic pill and within five and half hours I lost four pound. My blood pressure went down and my headaches went away. Also being human my spirits were higher and I was quite happy to see the scale move.

Well, well it is Girl Scout Cookie time and all the things that I thought I had learned have flown right out the window. Self control, portion control, gone and the what the hell effect came flying in like a bomb. Even as I sat there eating that whole box of peanut butter patties I knew that there was no justifying it. But all the old excuses just kept running thru my head like a rerun. They won't be here tomorrow to tempt me. I ate four so what does it matter if I eat the rest. I'll just walk a few extra minutes because they only come once a year. The only thing that in my mind that made it better was that my skinny girlfriend did the same thing and she justified it for both of us by saying "you know that there isn't that many in a box any more and they are so small also." Then the next day I called another girlfriend and she made the comment that she was so uncomfortable and them proceeded to tell me that she ate too many Girl Scout cookies because they were sooo good. So through this whole thing I am glad to learn that I am not the only one to lose self control over Girl Scout cookies and next year I will just make a donation and tell them to take the cookies to the homeless shelter.

The last two weeks I have fallen by the way side and not have been as faithful as I should be. It is very easy to fall back into old habits. Being fat is just plain easier, no work, no effort, and no commitment. I have found my self saying oh a couple Dortios won't hurt, a extra serving of carbs won't make that much of a difference. But we all know that it does. It would be so easy not to have written all this and let everyone think that I am doing everything right. But being human everyone knows that the reality of things is that I have slipped up and will probably do it again. I have been so depressed about the fluid retention that I have let this get in the way of being sensible and doing what I need to do to continue losing weight. I am up nine pounds in one week. This has been an issue my whole life of up down, up down in weight. The yo-yo syndrome. I have become the champion of yo yo dieting. I could easily say that in my life time I have lost over 1000 pounds and possibly more.

I am still doing the tread mill five days a week and even walked around the block the other day. But I have not been doing true balanced blocks. Still eating fresh fruits and veggies, but not measuring them out like I should be. Some where in the last two weeks I have loss the portion control. So I need to regroup and move forward again and start thinking like a thin person. I deserve to be thinner and to do the things that I want to do. My inner thin person is crying to get out; she so desperately wants to be all that she can be and to be free of the quilt of being fat. Who would ever think that the issue of being too fat or too thin could carry so much pain, hurt, and guilt. There is so many times on this journey that I find myself crying. It is a cleansing of the soul and ones inner peace. Then there is the fact that as human beings we are harder on ourselves then we should be. We should be thinking would we be this hard on our friends? No, so then we should give ourselves a break and give ourselves the encouragement that we would give a friend. Easier said then done thou.

I don't know what it is about April and May that makes my arthritis act up. I am so sore, stiff, and my bones snap, crackle, and pop more than a bowl of Rice Krispies. I had to have Tyler help me last night to get up off a chair. This is something that he has not had to help me with since I have lost the weight. My left knee is becoming very painful and has started to catch and has now gone out on me twice when walking. I have found myself thinking how to avoid walking and planning the shortest distance to do something. Something I have not done since getting my artificial knee. This is not good! I am so afraid that I will not have the weight off before having to have surgery on this knee.

Still having issues with the water weight gain and the doctor has changed my medicine again. Since the scale has not been moving in the right direction at all for almost a month I feel not only have I let myself down, but all those who have been impressed by my changes and success to this point.

At some point on this journey I feel that I need to reflect on my childhood and what it was like being the biggest kid in class. This is very painful to write about and expose about one's self and will bring many tears while writing. I was the tallest at one point along with another girl named Barb. I wouldn't really consider myself obese when I was younger. I was just a big kid. But kids are so cruel. I would wake up everyday and hope that things would be different at school. First my day would start out that I was the last one to be one picked up by the bus. No one wanted me to sit with them. So I would have to walk the whole length of the bus asking if I could sit with them only to be turned down and humiliated. I would always end up sitting with the girl who had a hygiene problem. The other kids would laugh and make comments about how I was too fat to sit any where. Then I would arrive at school to no friends and no one to talk to too. Only to be called the too familiar names on the play ground, fatty, fat so, lard butt, and many more. Then to be humiliated once again every day in the lunch room because no one wanted me to sit by them their either. To always be the last one picked to play on a team. They always acted like my weight was contagious. I am so very thankful for having one really good friend during this time and her named was Bobbie. She made things bearable for me. I was always picked on about my clothes. Considering now that I am 44 that gives you a time frame of when I grew up. That would be the 70's.

Back then there were no large size stores, especially for kids. Clothes were impossible then to find that would be nice, let alone have some style to them. Any thing that would fit me looked like grandmas clothes. Or to be more precise I would call them grandma grunt clothes. I was never in style with any of my clothes. I really believe that is one of the reasons that I started to sew. Then there was gym in junior high being so embarrassing and almost unbearable at times. Gym teachers were unmerciful to the over weight kids. Let alone the fact that back then we were made to take showers and were herded through them like cattle, nothing private about them at all. Everything and anything exposed for all to see. At this age one is trying to find their identity and dealing with ones self image and then also have to deal with everyone staring at you in the locker room. It is bad enough when kids call you names about your weight and now the locker room has given them more ammunition. They now have seen every bump and lump of fat on your body that you so desperately tried to hide with your clothes. Plus any stretch marks that you may have had. Also with me I had extremely large breast that were an issue, which I later had reduced. Lucky for me I had a good self esteem about myself and was able to have some very good friends through high school who truly liked me for me and seen past the fat.

Another thing about being fat is the issue with some doctors. You can go to the doctor say for an infected finger and some how before you leave you get the big lecture about your weight. First off don't these doctors think that I know I am fat and I know that I have or will have issues because of this? Secondly this type of behavior makes it so that we don't even want to go to the doctor for anything. These doctors try to contribute all our health problems to our weight. Thirdly it is really sad when a doctor refuses to treat you because of your weight. I have had this happen several times to myself. These doctors will say something like "When you lose some weight come back and we can discuss your options then." Hello, there is a problem now that is why one is at the doctor in the first place. I am fat and that is who I am so you need to deal with me as I am now I would tell them. Just because I am fat doesn't mean that my issues should not be treated or brushed off. At times I would have to be very assertive or blunt and ask them; "How would you treat me if I was a thin person?" Sometimes this would throw them off guard and I would get a more realistic treatment, instead of the suggestion of weight loss surgery. Several times I had to find a different doctor that did not have an issue with me being over weight.

I have been in a panic because my tread mill is on the blink. It will be five to seven business days before the part gets here. So I have been walking a half mile around the neighborhood with my son at night which hasn't been too bad and also a half mile in the morning. I do have to stop at times and let the cramps pass in my feet and hips. It really has been a pleasure taking these walks with my son. My next goal is to walk the track at school and then back home. That will be a mile and hopefully then do it again in the evening. Time will tell. Well, time did tell and the track was a no go. My feet and hips cramped so bad I was afraid that I wasn't going to make it back home. It sure would have been embarrassing to have had to call the police just to be picked up and taken me home. I guess that is why I like the tread mill. I can stop and start as my body allows me. But I sure do like the walks outside thou.

It is April 20th and I have not stepped on the scale now for thirteen days. I am afraid of what it will show and then be reduced to tears again. But I will have to buck up and just remember that I am weighing myself to keep on track and it is only a tool to guide me. To remember that it is just there to help me work harder and not get depressed over it. So now that I have given myself the pep talk, it is off to the clinic to have a one on one with the metal beast of numbers. Well the scale did move two pounds which is better than nothing and I will take it.

For Easter I made myself a dress, the first thing that I have sewn for myself since the weight loss. I have to be honest here and say I was actually a little nervous about this because I wasn't sure what size I was going to be. I felt like I was sewing for the first time. It was the first time in years that I did not have to enlarge the pattern. It was fun and strange at the same time that I just had to lay the pattern on the material and just cut it out. No fudging to make it fit or no skimping just to get it out. So I used less material and it cost me less. I also made myself a waist jacket for the dress instead of the long jacket to cover my butt. This was a daring thing for me to do, because I am always trying to cover things up. I am going to make myself some summer tops now and shorts. I can't believe that I will be wearing shorts again.

I think that I found out what some of the problem has been with all the weight gain. Fish oil pills. Researching on the internet I found that they can cause weight gain, increase sugar levels, stomach upset, headaches and more. I stopped taking them and after two days I did not wake up with swollen eyelids and my ankles were no longer full of fluid either and I feel better. I don't feel as stiff either since not having all that fluid on me. Also my nagging headache is gone.

There is no way to write this without being brutally descriptive and honest. It is not a pretty picture nor is it funny. But since losing weight my abdomen folds are becoming more of a pain then before. The folds are looser so they are trapping more moisture and causing some pretty sore areas. These areas will get so fire engine red, and sore that sometimes it even hurts to walk. They will burn so that it will feel like it is on fire at times. Oh, by the way don't forget the strong foul offensive odor these things can also cause. I have to take a wash cloth and fold it just right so that the skin is not on skin so that it can heal, just for another one to pop out some where else. Another reason I am getting more of these areas is because I am exercising and sweating more than I use too. Yes, I take showers everyday, but it still doesn't stop these nasty things from happening. It is one of those embarrassing things that a fat person lives with and hopes that no one will ever know about it. The tears are flowing as I write this because this really is the bearing of my soul. But I want people to understand that being fat has some issues that no one would ever think of. No one wishes or wants to be obese. Being fat is and can be very embarrassing, humiliating, and unbearable at times and for some a very desperate situation. These feelings come from our own feelings of guilt and from how people treat us. Being fat has so many hidden secrets with tears and pain. Some of the pain and humiliation comes from fellow obese people who give obese people a bad rap by wearing clothes to small for them. I am not one to cast stones, but even being obese myself I find it very disgusting when I see men and women's stomachs hanging below their shirts for the whole world to see. Or when a women a tries to squish herself into half shirts and their jeans look they were put on while lying on the bed holding their breath. So then their fat rolls are flopping over their jeans. Being heavy doesn't mean that we can't dress nice. But we also need to be realistic and know that the public doesn't want to see our fat, especially when we live in such a thin orientated world. I am also smart enough to realize that we now live in a world where people have the "I don't give a damn attitude", but that doesn't mean we can't have pride in how we look.

Since I have started losing weight I have been doing a lot of reading about weight loss, exercising, health issues and so much more. I have always known that the world worships sliminess and fears the obese. But I have never known till now to what degree we are considered sub humans. To many people obesity symbolizes one's inability not to have self control, huge appetites, and not having the ability to maintain personal health. Fat people are often perceived as lazy, failures, stupid, smelly and dirty. Because of this it some how seems that it has become socially acceptable to be rude to obese people. It is like we are to have no emotions or feelings and just accept it. I am neither lazy, a failure, stupid, smelly or dirty. I am a professional, well kept retired nurse who runs her own business. Has society called over weight celebrities lazy, under achievers, dirty, smelly, stupid or a failure.

This next section is taken from a website just to show what other people think about obese people and how cruel they are. fatpeoplearestupid.com/archives/2004/10/index.html:

Here we go again! Now two fat women are suing Southwest Airlines because Southwest decided what other airlines should have instituted long ago; A your too fat so you pay double policy. Fat people across America want to boycott the airline and I say, PLEASE! More room for me. Lawsuits site that these women were singled out, abused, and humiliated. I want to go on record saying, so what! If you have ever sat next to a size 22 woman you know what I mean. The only one being abused is the passenger sitting next to the size 22 behemoth. When are these people going to stop playing the victim and start becoming a proactive member of society? Fat people don't ever take into consideration other individuals discomfort with their fat rolls spilling over the arm rest and into unsuspecting passengers lap and don't let me remind you that when you're that big. YOU STINK! And you stink even more when you're on that stupid Atkins diet. I am getting sick of fat people whining about how people treat them. They have the ability to not to be fat; no one is force feeding you Big Mac's by the truckload. Oh, that's right you don't really eat that much and you're fat because someone else is eating for you. Who the hell do you think you're kidding? I want to send a message to Southwest Airlines, if they can keep all fat people off the plane, I'll pay double. Some may call this mean spirited, uncaring, and wrong. Well I pronounce to you that I do care and it may be mean but there has to be an end to this ridiculous rise in obesity. If it takes an airline to just say no to fat passengers than so be it. I say get your food gorging, lazy ass moving in a direction that will help you fit I into an Airline seat. Posted by Rocco. I think that there is nothing more for me to say about this article. It says it all and leaves one feeling the disgust and cruelty. This is just one site of many that feel this way. But I do need to make a comment about the hygiene. Most heavy people are very self conscious about odors and very meticulous about their hygiene in general.

After reading that article it just amazes me how our society has no tolerance for obesity. Yet it accepts body piercing in places that shouldn't be. It accepts our teens wearing spiked dog collars, with hair any color imaginable that isn't a natural color and wearing their jeans to their knees with their under wear sticking out.

I happen to catch Law and Order the other night when the lawyer tried using obesity as a defensive to murder. I think that was ridiculous using obesity like that, I can see why some people complain that heavy people are not being responsible for themselves and using their fat as an accuse.

Well there is another surprise on this journey. Lately I have had my glasses off more than on and the reason being is that my eyes have gotten better. My eye doctor said that is because my labs have gotten better and I am healthier.

The scale had not moved for over two weeks, but still maintaining what I have lost thou. So I am switching some things with my diet. I am now having a soy protein shake for breakfast and lunch with a meal for supper with a one or two block snack before bed. Hopefully that will jump start my system again.

I wore out my tread mill in four months. It will cost over $300.00 to get it fixed. So for now it will be walking outside and save my pennies. Hopefully I will be able to have it fixed by the time snow flies. If not I guess I'll have to get a pair of snow shoes. They are probably a lot cheaper. But then I would have to get a snow suit and the other entire garb that goes with it, and then I would be cold so, that I would have to drink hot chocolate. That would then defeat the walk, so in the long run it might not be any cheaper.

May third and I weighed myself this morning and the scale just won't budge. No matter how many times I said, "Jeanne the scale is just a tool," the tears just kept coming. I so want to be thinner. Nobody can even begin to feel how I feel. Right now I feel desperate and like a failure. I am disappointed and feel like I am at a dead end. The tears today just won't stop. It would be so easy just to say to hell with it and throw a pizza in the oven. But I won't and I am not giving in, I won't, I just won't. I want this too bad and it is my life to live this way. I have once again asked God to help me as I am sobbing at the keyboard.

I am now having so much pain in my left knee and pain from my lower back which I really feel in my leg. The pain in my leg is so bad that I have a hard time falling asleep and it wakes me up. I have been taking my pain pills and a muscle relaxant and they just barely take the edge off. I am hoping that the chiropractor will help. If not then I have a new issue to deal with. I have had back surgery once all ready. If there would be a need for surgery again I most definitely have to have the weight off.

Last night I went out to eat with some friends and I over ate and ate too many carbs. So this morning I woke up with a headache and I wished I could of puked, I felt so awful. So as humans do we just do this to remind ourselves of why we have made these life changes to eat healthlier. Because if we do this, for that reason, I have learnt my lesson again until the next reminder binge.

Since losing weight I have a lot more energy and have enjoyed using that energy doing gardening again. For the past few years I have not done any gardening because being honest it was difficult moving around and I had no energy. My son is building me two raised flower gardens in the front yard so that it won't irritate my arthritic joints. When it is all done my yard will be full of bright color and blooms.

Well I have been at a stand still for sometime and have to realize that my body has adjusted to its new life style. So now I have to start doing different things to get my body to lose again. So I am going to try counting calories now for something different. I am also going to try some weight lifting. Not sure if I will be able to do it with my joints or not but going to give it a try and see what happens. So I went to the gym last night and looked around and I am going to give it a try for a week and see what my joints think of it. Stepped on the scale while there and I have lost a pound, yeah.

Well these last two weeks I have done something's that I would of never considered before, let alone doing them. For one I walked a half mile for United Cerebral Palsy in the rain and cold. Secondly I joined Gold's Gym. Tyler is more excited about this then I am. It can be embarrassing at a gym because for one being fat you can't fit on all the weight machines, so once again trying to fit into a thin world. Secondly there are mirrors all over so there is no avoiding the truth that you are fat and no matter how thin my brain thinks I am, the mirrors do not lie as I sit there on a machine with my fat spilling all over with the truth staring me in the face. The funny thing is that my mirrors at home don't show that side of me to myself. So I continue to work out with disgust as I watch myself in these mirrors with some skinny toned chick next to me. Working out at the gym does have one exercising more thou. I now work out for an hour three to four days a week and walk the other days.

It is six months into this new life style and I am doing okay with it. The scale is still not moving down, but it is not going up either. I am hoping that by going to the gym I will get the scale moving again. I don't think that people realize what it really takes to lose weight. It is not just counting calories, carbs, fats, proteins, exercising, and drinking a lot of water. It is exercising the right way to gain muscle and not lose it. It is eating the right carbs, fats, and proteins in the right portions. Our bodies are a very defined piece of equipment that really has a mind of its own so to say. We have to keep changing things around all the time to keep our bodies guessing and not getting use to what we are doing. Losing weight can be a full time job in itself.

Since going to the gym my clothes feel loser and believe it or not I have some muscle when I flex my arm. One pound away from hitting the 55 pound mark again. I have also lost an inch on my waist.

Also I got a part time job so now I will be juggling that with the gym. I will also have to be very careful not to slip back into the old habits of eating the wrong way because it is easier or because I am too tired to cook. Since working I am noticing that I feel more tired and sore.

Even thou I am still obese I now find myself looking at other obese people and thinking, Oh, my God I need to work harder at this change of life. Because I am not going to look like that any more as I am gazing at very large obese man and women. I also now find myself watching what other people are eating and thinking do they know what they are doing to themselves.

I am still going to the gym facing the brutally and truth of the mirrors. The scale is still not moving up or down so to speak. In one day the scale went up seven pounds and I did not freak out this time nor did it bother me. I can weigh in at the beginning of my work out and then after my work out and ten minutes in the sauna I can weigh myself again and the scale has dropped two pounds, so I know it is all water. I am still so desperately waiting for the scale to start moving in a down ward direction.

I am also walking at a faster rate with a one notch incline on the tread mill. Some days I feel that I am walking so fast that my fat is causing friction. That I am waiting for the smoke to start bellowing out from my thighs. I do know that the gym is building muscle thou. My posture is better, I actually feel taller. My stomach is more toned and I have increased the amount of weights.

Well, with all this water weight gain up and down I have lost probably close to a thirty pounds. Too bad it wasn't all fat! At least the scale is not going up at this time. One of the trainers at the gym stated that they have had people at a plateau for 6 months or more. That is really depressing to me. So on that note I still continue to go to the gym and eat better.

On this journey I am still in awe of things. I worked out side in the yard today for two whole hours! It was so awesome that I was able to do it for one thing. Secondly I did not get out of breath or felt uncomfortable doing it. It is so amazing what our body's can do when the foundation is stronger. Since gaining muscle my body as a whole functions so much smoother with less pain. I actually feel stronger as a whole, and mentally as well. I am still waiting for the scale to move. But in all I am happy because of how good I feel about myself and that I am able to do things again that I truly enjoy such as gardening and working in the yard. Some things I have not been able to do for at least four to five years now. Just the fact that I was able to do these activities was a feat in its self, let alone feeling great after wards. Activities that we all take for grant it. So once again I thank God for his gift of my life and the ability to live it. For only God and myself know what today truly meant to me. There are no words to describe it.

Well, I did over do it in the yard yesterday. By last night I could hardly move and real stiff this morning. So I will have to watch how much I do and then quit, no matter how good I am feeling at the time.

Today is June eighteenth and the scale still hasn't moved in the direction I would like. It keeps going up and down those five to ten pounds of water that I keep gaining and losing. I am really getting discouraged. There are days that it is more and more tempting to go back to my old ways of eating because it is easier and more convenient.

Also the fact that there is no work or will power needed to eat the other way either. I really did have a bad night last night. I was eating a lot of carbs and ended up with a terrific carb headache to boot. This must have been my reminder binge to keep me in line.

I now find myself thinking ok if I could only lose 50 pounds I will settle for that and be happy. I keep shortening my goals because I don't see them happening any more. Sitting here sobbing, my inner skinny self is screaming I want out and yet I don't seem to be able to know how to do it any more. I am eating right, and exercising to my limitations because if I go over it then I pay for it for days afterwards. I feel like I am stuck and can't get out. I ask God everyday to help me and let it be his will that I lose more weight. I am to a point where I am ready to throw the towel in with tears streaming down my cheeks. This is so dam hard. Nobody knows my pain and hurt, or what it is like to be fat for me and so want to be thinner.

Somehow to be able to fit in to this thin orientated world that society has created and be in the "norm" of things. No longer having to navigate through a thin person's world of verbal abuse and cruelty. To be able to wear what ever you want. To buy clothes where you want and not have to buy them at a fat store, where the selection is not always the greatest if any at all. For some reason manufactures think that fat people should be covered in flowers and gaudy designs with sequins across their breast. Does one ever see smaller size clothes in the designs that they make fat clothes in? No, of course not because thin people won't be caught dead in them! To be able to go any where, sit in a chair there and fit. Not to worry whether it is going to break or not. To quit hearing people say you can lose weight if you want to, you just aren't trying hard enough. These people will never know how hard it is. They will never be able to comprehend what it is like. To always having to be conscious of what I eat or don't eat. Food isn't food any more; it's calories, carbs, fats, and proteins. If I have a dessert, it isn't that was a nice treat. Now it is that is another fifteen minutes more of extra exercising.

Well today is June twenty second and I did some measuring and what a nice surprise, the tape measure has gone up in some areas. I have gained an inch on my thighs, my arms and my chest. This is a good thing because it explains why the scale hasn't been moving. I have gained muscle mass and we all know that it weighs more than fat. I also lost another inch on my waist. When I stepped on the scale I have lost a pound. Also on the tread mill I can walk at a speed of 2.5 for a while with a 3.0 incline for about five minutes on and off.

I have really come to a cross roads here. The scale just won't budge and plain old math says that I am taking in as many calories that I am burning. For one I can't drop my calorie count any farther, because then I would kick in the starvation mode. Secondly I can't work out any longer or harder with my exercises because then my arthritis has a fit and then I can't do anything for few days. My left knee and feet have gotten worse since I went back to work part time. I am sore all the time again and especially at night again. My toes are numb and my feet hurt gain to the point that I want to cry when I walk. My left knee has been catching and going out on me now. The other morning I had to walk with my cane, because my knee was so unstable. I was walking outside and almost took a nose dive when it went out on me. My doctor had no answers for me either.

I surely do not want to gain what I have lost! Just if there really was that magic pill or diet that really worked, it would make this so much easier.

I have been working outside a lot more now this year, because I can move easier and have more energy. My flower garden out front is finished and looks so beautiful. It felt so good again to feel that accomplishment of having something grow and have people comment on how nice it looks.

Well on this journey I have taken a detour. I haven't been to the gym over three weeks and I haven't been following the portion control too well. Still eating the right things but a little more than I should be. It is amazing how fast your muscles go back to the way they were before exercising. I can feel it in my clothes, so I went back to the gym today and it felt good. My muscles wanted to retaliate a little, but I gave them no slack. The scale was only up six pounds, it could have been worse.

Where does one begin? No one ever said that life would not be easy nor did it come with an instruction manual. I have had to do some real soul searching of late and really don't like some of the things that I am realizing. One I will always be fat and my inner skinny self will always be there, but deeply hidden in the fat. I have given it my all and it is just not in the cards for me to be thin. I will continue to be unhappy with my body and all the grief that it gives. I will not look at this as a failure but as a stepping stone to learning. Still hoping in my heart that the world will realize that life is about seeing people for who they are in the inside, and that the out side is only the shell that holds the heart.

So as I come to the end of this journey I only hope that this journal has helped some people see the other side. I want all heavy people to be proud of who they are and what they are, and to realize and know that you have to be happy with in yourself. To remember that all the criticism, negative and rudeness comes from people who are thin and have no idea what our world is like. The thin people who obsessive about their weight understand. These people are the ones that eat what ever they want when they want. They are the ones that do not have to think what a calorie or carb is let alone to try and keep count of them. They probably don't even think about exercising let alone doing it. They are uneducated in their thinking that all heavy people have large appetites and have no self control. We all know unless they were to walk our shoes and wear our fat they will never truly know the other side. If I had one wish it would be that every thin person had to wear a fat suit for one month, count calories and carbs, exercise, and to feel what I do everyday of my life. To feel, understand, and realize that it isn't always about our choices or desires.

It has been over a year now of making my life changes. Yes I am still unhappy with my weight, so on that note I am going to take another journey. With some soul searching I have decided to make yet another life change. With this change I will have to be even more dedicated and really change my whole why of thinking and looking at food. As a society we have really come to eat just to eat and not to eat to survive. I have chosen to have the Lap Band surgery. I have chosen this surgery over other methods because I feel that it is less evasive, safer, and one is not disturbing the natural flow of digestion. With this procedure, exercising, learning to eat only to survive I feel that my inner thin self will be able to emerge. I will some day be in the "norm" of things. I know that this is going to be very difficult and a hard journey. I am not kidding myself one bit that it will easy at any point. But now where does it say that life is easy. There is always going to be sacrifices or things that one has to give up for the ultimate goal.

This surgery will change my whole life in every aspect. At this point I don't see myself going out to eat after surgery. As I sit here and think I know that I truly enjoy sitting down with a cup of coffee and eating breakfast. It is not the act of eating it self that is satisfying, it is the mental eating. Thinking of all the things that I will have to change in my head and realize that I only need the three cups of food a day to survive. Also knowing myself as well as I do, I will have to work very hard with the dietician on meals so that I am getting what I need for nutrition. Because I already know that I would just grab a cup of cottage cheese and call it good. So as the whole process begins I am just taking it one day at a time and getting myself and my mind frame where it will need to be for the rest of my life. I will need my God, family and friends more then I have ever needed them for support.

Well it is now five years later and I am still fat. I decided not to have the lap band surgery. I did more research and decided that this was not the answer either. I ended up with too many fears and doubts. Because so many people after this surgery end up with long life digestive problems and infections. Some have lived shortened lives even with the weight loss and others have gain weight back.

But my journey five years ago was not a complete waste. I still eat the majority of good foods over junk food. I still don't eat a sweet after a meal. I kept ten pounds off out of the fifty I had lost and I still prefer fruits over breads. And yes exercise is still the key to feeling good. No matter what the exercise is it better than no exercise.

But I have more health issues and the arthritis has not been kind. Had another back surgery this summer and ended up with some slight residuals. My right elbow now keeps me from doing the simplest things, such as washing dishes, and scrubbing the stove off to name just a few things. Also during this time frame exercise has become next to impossible. Worked with a physical therapist for a while and it was so hard to do the things that she wanted me to do. The arthritis has made so many more things difficult. Once again not my choice or desire not to do the things that she wanted me to do. She asked me a question; "with your physical limitations keeping you from doing things are you happy with your weight?" I need to answer that by asking myself this question;" I am happy with the things that I can no longer do because of the arthritis, definitely not." So knowing that the weight comes partly from my physical limitations, I am happy with who I am. Thus my weight is a part of who I am. But some days it is hard to accept the weight, so in reality I do not like how I look and will still cry at times because of it.

I am now going to the gym three days a week to exercise in the pool. It feels so good to be moving and doing movements that I can not do on land. For example being able to walk without a limp, something so simple yet taken for granted.

Society as a whole is still getting heavier, yet the mind set is still in the thin mode of thinking. People are still mocking obesity, being cruel making fun of the heavy person and don't think that this is a disease. It is still cheaper to buy junk food than to buy healthily food. Restaurants are still offering their meals to be made bigger for a few pennies more. Thus the general public doesn't even know what a normal portion of food looks like any more. They still think that heavy people are lazy, slobs, and have no self discipline.

My inner skinny self is still there hidden with in the fat folds. I live one day at a time and know that in my heart I gave it a good try. I have decided that if I can walk on my own and wipe my own butt it is a good day.

Still hoping that the world sees people for who they are and not how they look. Hoping that people can see pass the skin, fat, warts, and deformities of others to see the inner beauty of people and what they have to offer the world. I would like to believe that if everyone would look deep within themselves they would find the heart that God had intended them to have. So no matter what your personal issues may be, just remember never take the simple things for grant it, always appreciate the things that you can do, tell your family and friends that you love them, don't be afraid to hug someone, and thank God for all your blessings. To remember that Obesity has no limits to age, gender, race, creed, the famous, the poor or the wealthy.